Contents

D1329232

Acknowledgements

Thanks are given to Helen Jones, Alison Williams and especially Gill Frances, without whom this publication would not have happened. Thanks also to John Mitchell, for his help in researching policy and practice in the Department du Nord, France.

Special thanks to Jane Hobden for her speedy, careful editing.

Introduction

Children and young people who are looked after are among the most socially excluded of all young people. They are reported to have greater health needs than their peers, yet are less likely to receive adequate health care and treatment or be supported in developing their knowledge and skills in making decisions that promote health and well-being. They need to be cared for in a setting that actively promotes health and well-being for children, young people as well as staff and carers.

The National Healthy Care Standard programme is being developed to promote health and well-being for looked after children and young people, and those leaving care, by building on existing good practice, partnerships and policies. To inform this process, the National Children's Bureau carried out two literature reviews – one from a national perspective (Howell and Chambers 2001 unpublished), the other from an international perspective (Olle and Madge 2001 unpublished). The international review also includes information collected from specific individuals in different countries working in the residential care field, and a small-scale survey of policy and practice. Both reviews are brought together in this report, which examines the health needs of looked after children and sets out current standards and guidance in England. It also identifies existing work, and provides health promotion models for the development of future practice. The study of practice in other countries serves to mirror and reinforce priorities for practice in England. However it also highlights some differences, perhaps the most important of which relates to the status, training and role of child care workers.

Both reviews emphasise the need for continuity and consistency in health care, and conclude that health care should be seen from the perspective of well-being rather than from the narrow disease model from which it is currently often viewed. This wider perspective encompasses all aspects of a child's life and experiences and provides a better basis for promoting a young person's health and well-being.

This publication builds the underpinning evidence for the National Healthy Care Standard (NHCS) Programme, and is the first document in a series of Guidance papers for the national roll out of NHCS.

NHCS is a national programme to promote the health and well-being of looked after children. The NHCS programme aims to ensure that children and young people who are looked after have access to:

- an environment that promotes children and young people's health and well-being with trained and supported carers and within the wider community;
- effective health assessments and treatment, excellent health services and care;
- opportunities to develop the personal social and life skills to care for their health and well-being, now and in the future.

Factors affecting the health of looked after children and young people

Poor physical and mental health

> 'One of the biggest things that came out of the report was health and like a lot of young people have got ill health, I mean you've got physical and mental, a lot of young people I interviewed were turning to drugs and things like that because they just couldn't cope because they were depressed all the time ... everybody I interviewed was on drugs at some time after leaving care, ended up underweight, just basically because they couldn't afford to eat ... because they had to pay bills ... I think what's needed in my own opinion is some sort of health education ... '
>
> *(SAVE THE CHILDREN 1995)*

The physical and mental health of children in care is too often very poor in comparison to that of their peers, with higher levels of substance misuse (Department of Health 1997a), significantly higher rates of teenage pregnancy than for the non-care population (Corlyon and McGuire 1997, Brodie, Berridge and Beckett 1997, Biehal and others 1992 and 1995), and a much greater prevalence of mental health problems (Bamford and Wolkind 1988, McCann and others 1996, Buchanan 1999, Arcelus, Bellerby and Vostanis 1999, Dimigen and others 1999, Richardson and Joughin 2000).

England is not alone in recognising the issue of poor health among looked after children. There is increasing awareness in most countries that this group of young people have high rates of poor overall health. Research in Canada, for example, has highlighted how many children enter care with poor health (Cain and Barth 1990 *mentioned in* Kufeldt and others 2000). These children often have undetected and untreated health problems, including an undocumented and poor history of immunisation, as well as problems with vision, hearing and growth. In Western Australia, Clare and Clare (2000) comment that research literature shows that there are difficulties in adequately meeting the physical and emotional health needs of children placed in out-of-home settings. Welfare professionals involved in a study in Perth were concerned about evidence of younger children being poorly nourished, lacking routine and generally neglected in placements.

The rates of self harm and high risk behaviour among those in the care setting, particularly young people in secure accommodation, is another indicator of poor mental and emotional well-being (Shaw and Who Cares? Trust 1998). Such behaviour is often considered attention-seeking, a coping mechanism, or a young person's behaviour being out of control. Stewart-Brown in Buchanan and Hudson (2000) provides a model of well-being based on the child's need to be parented 'with respect, empathy and genuineness', so enabling them to experience well-being and develop ways of relating to others that enhances their own and others' well-being (Appendix 1). Absence of respectful parenting leads to distress and destructive and unhelpful ways of coping, including violence and criminality (Buchanan and Hudson 2000). Lack of appropriate, consistent parenting may contribute to behaviour difficulties and in some cases referral to Child and Adolescent Mental Health Services (CAMHS) and resultant pathologising of the young person.

The poor physical and mental health of young people in or leaving care has concerned some practitioners and policy makers for many years. Barbara Kahan (1989) cited the conclusions of the 1984 Short Report on the failures of corporate parents to respond adequately to the health needs of the children in their care:

> 'Because a child in care lacks one single person intimately familiar with his medical history, symptoms which normal caring parents would be in a position to observe and interpret may go unnoticed, so that they may suffer from non-acute but serious problems such as hearing or sight defects or other long-standing conditions such as asthma or diabetes. Younger children in particular may miss out on the proper series of inoculations and dental treatment may be unduly intermittent.'
>
> *(KAHAN 1989)*

Kahan expressed the hope that the Children Act 1989 would significantly improve the health outcomes for children in care, not least because of the greater emphasis within the Act on preventive work with children and families. However a series of more recent reports indicate that improvements in health indicators and outcomes have failed to materialise (Saunders and Broad 1997, Utting 1997, Acheson 1998, House of Commons Health Committee 1998, Skuse and Ward 1999, and Wyler 2000).

Greater awareness of mental health

The Royal College of Psychiatrists has acknowledged the need to promote greater awareness of mental health issues and concerns amongst those caring for and working with looked after children, by the publication of a book on the subject. According to Richardson and Joughin, writing for the Royal College:

> 'The most common disorders which these young people and those caring for them suffer from include: anxiety, fears and depression, conduct disorder and

attachment disorder. A smaller group develop serious mental illness, such as schizophrenia and bipolar affective disorder, with psychotic symptoms (which may not always be identified) in the early stages. The experience of early sexual abuse and violence may predispose some victims to become abusers themselves or to fear that they will do so. Very often despair about their lives or the need to draw attention to their dire predicament leads to suicidal attempts and self-harming behaviour.'

(RICHARDSON AND JOUGHIN 2000)

The authors point out that health problems rarely come singly. A complex and inter-linked set of risk-taking or offending behaviours involving self harm, running away, misuse of drugs and alcohol, unsafe sex and frequent change of partners, as well as vulnerability to sexual exploitation and abuse, may all present as the external symptoms of low self-esteem and mental distress. At the same time they point out that many social workers and other carers are rightly wary of labelling young people with psychiatric diagnoses. The stigmatising of young people in the care system – the 'mad, bad and sad' label so resented by many who are or have been in care – has undoubtedly contributed to negative expectations of them, which as the authors point out may further damage already vulnerable self-esteem:

'There is an understandable fear that this process further damages the frail self-esteem of young people and that it creates negative expectations in them and those educating and taking care of them, which becomes self-fulfilling.'

(IBID)

It is important to note that most people working with looked after children are largely untrained in matters specifically relating to mental health, despite the fact that they have to respond to, and address the needs of, some very vulnerable and emotionally damaged young people.

Failing to meet the needs of specific groups of looked after children

The care system is also failing to meet the needs of children with disabilities. Research shows that service providers all too often ignore the disabled young person's right to have a say in their care. This, along with confusion about funding and provision, results in unmet health care and social needs (Morris 1995). The transition from children's to adult services and/or 'independence' is even more unsatisfactory, described by some young people with disabilities as like 'hurtling into a void'.

'... a lack of information is one of the key barriers identified by young disabled people ... if young people with health care needs generally find that information

about their condition is an important part of becoming an independent adult, then this increases the importance of their autonomous relationship with medical and other professionals. It means that finding out about the condition or illness, the needs associated with it and the best way of meeting those needs, is an important part of the transition to adulthood for young people with health care and support needs.'

(MORRIS 1999)

Children from minority ethnic backgrounds may suffer particular discrimination within the care system. Training on the particular health needs of minority groups is *'woefully inadequate'* in the view of many practitioners (Mather 2000a).

'For a child in the care system who has been separated from family and home for some time, it is too easy to assume that cultural issues no longer matter. It is also easy to make erroneous assumptions about which cultural issues are important to others. Medical practitioners need to open up to the importance of cultural issues but be led by the child and her or his parents in recognising the issues most relevant to them.'

(IBID)

In another recent study, young black disabled people registered loneliness as a significant issue when living independently, and complained of a lack of informal support or chances for them to meet other young black disabled people and to share experiences (Bignall and Butt 2000).

According to one study, despite the *'wealth of information'* about looked after young people there are *'major gaps'* in our knowledge on health issues with regard to gender and ethnicity. More empirical knowledge is needed to underpin interventions (Aggleton, Hurry and Warwick 2000).

In other countries, belonging to a minority ethnic group is also associated with increased disadvantage in many respects. However it is unclear what possible lessons could be learned. One American study found that both Caucasian and Hispanic children in foster care in California had higher rates of death and injury than their counterparts in the general population but no such differences were found for those from African American backgrounds (Barth and Blackwell 1998). A related study found that Caucasian young people were more likely than those from either African American or Hispanic backgrounds to be referred for or use psychotherapy services (Garland and Besinger 1997).

Lack of continuity of care

In 1998, the then Chief Medical Officer Sir Donald Acheson conducted an independent inquiry into inequalities in health. After citing numerous risk factors and poor health indicators relating to looked after children, he summed up the situation as follows:

'... looked-after children are a key target group for policies related to education, employment and housing, and to health related behaviour ... however they are further disadvantaged in their access to health care, both preventative and therapeutic. Their increased mobility may result in fragmentation of, and delay in, service delivery, including assessment of, and provision for, their educational and health needs, including health promotion.'

(ACHESON 1998)

The physical and mental health problems of children in care and leaving care may be deeply rooted in their pre-care experience and circumstances, the very factors which led to their coming into care, but the worrying issue for care providers is the evidence that the period 'in care' can actually exacerbate rather than reduce existing problems, and can even create new dangers:

'... far from remedying existing deficiencies ... periods in public care have further impaired the life chances of some children and young people because of poor educational achievement, uncorrected health problems and maladjustment.'

(DEPARTMENT OF HEALTH IN BUTLER AND PAYNE 1997)

Another recurring theme in the review is the significant gaps in the health records of children in care, with records failing to follow the child from placement to placement *as well as* the poor quality of records that do exist. The *Looking After Children: Assessment and Action Records*, launched by the Department of Health in 1995 have introduced a more consistent framework for social workers and health professionals (see page 15).

Lack of continuity in care was also highlighted by the international review. Canada, Australia and France all reported a lack of continuous preventative and routine health care for looked after children. None appeared to have a policy for referring children and young people to health facilities such as youth counselling, mental health and drug and alcohol services. In Australia, carers of younger children reported difficulties in obtaining a child's health history, either from the family or from the health and welfare system. Health checks are made at the discretion of individual case managers, and there is no policy for referring young people to health facilities such as youth counselling and mental health services.

In California, Karpilow and others (1998) concluded that children and young people in foster care often failed to receive preventive and consistent health services due to inadequate medical records and limited access to care. A specific problem in the US is related to Medi-Cal (managed care programme), which is geared to serving children and their families who continue to live in the same place and to see one provider. Hence it does not meet the needs of children in foster care who tend to be highly mobile. Accessing health care is particularly difficult for mobile foster children placed outside their county of origin. There were also no clear guidelines or state policy in California to guide the development of a system to meet the health needs of foster children (Karpilow and others 1998).

Changes in placement

The type of placement a young person has can have considerable implications for their health and health care. A Canadian study by Simard, Vachon and Berube (*mentioned in* Kufeldt and others 2000) showed that children living with relatives experience fewer health care problems than those in foster care. Frequent changes in placement and health care provision can be detrimental. Research in Canada (Kudeldt and others 2000) concludes that a lack of continuous, preventative and routine health services means that the health of looked after children often deteriorates with each placement. Children with complex and ongoing medical conditions, who require continuity in care, frequently receive emergency health care from an unknown doctor.

This Canadian study has also shown that changes in placement can lead to difficulties in coordinating the work of agencies, social workers, foster parents and medical personnel. The transfer of health care from parents to carers can also lead to the loss of factual and intuitive knowledge that a parent has from intimate daily contact with the child. The impact of this on the child is that pre-existing conditions may not be picked up and treated appropriately, and that appropriate follow up care, such as immunisations, may not be carried out.

Missing out on education and school-based health promotion

The severely disrupted educational patterns of many looked after children, together with their high rates of exclusion and truancy, mean that they may often miss out on school-based medical checks and health promotion work. Loss of self-esteem due to educational failure and exclusion can further impair emotional health and well-being. Poor emotional and psychological health and feelings of low self-esteem or abandonment can understandably lead to ill health, depression and/or the use of escape/coping mechanisms such as substance misuse:

'The effects of being in care were alarming for the majority of the young people. Most experienced great stress and insecurity which for many led to: a turning to drugs, alcohol or offending as a means of escape; and/or to stress related physical illnesses such as asthma; and/or to mental ill health, generally in the form of depression.'

(SAUNDERS AND BROAD 1997)

Assembling the data

Assessment and action records: the first year report

The *Looking After Children (LAC): Assessment and Action Records,* launched by the Department of Health in 1995, introduced a more consistent framework for social workers, in collaboration with others, to record and track essential information, including information about age-related assessments to prompt action at the appropriate stage. The assessment process covers wider aspects of development which impact on health, such as identity (including ethnic and cultural considerations), family and social relationships, education, emotional and behavioural development and self-care skills.

The report from the first year of data collection (Ward and Skuse 2001) does provide useful statistical evidence indicating the prevalence of certain health-related difficulties or conditions, amongst looked after children. The findings are based on a cohort study, which looks at the progress of 250 children, using data collected through the *Looking After Children* materials. Apart from specific medical conditions the data on 'Evidence of vulnerability' indicates relatively high levels of more general unmet health needs, with just over 50 per cent of the sample identified as having health and/or behavioural needs and nearly 75 per cent having problems with family and social relationships (see Appendix 2). The data similarly indicates a high rate of emotional and behavioural difficulties including conduct disorders, self-harming behaviour, relationship problems, inappropriate sexual behaviour, anxiety and bedwetting (see Appendix 2, Table 11). Ward and Skuse comment on the similar levels of conduct disorder to the data in the Oxfordshire study of McCann and others (1996). However Ward and Skuse found that other mental health problems such as depression or anxiety highlighted in the Oxfordshire study were much less evident from their data:

> *'The difference is more likely to be due to poor recording or lack of awareness than to genuine differences in behaviour patterns: while conduct disorders are hard to ignore, less obtrusive difficulties may be more easily overlooked. Much of the data concerning behavioural disorders was identified by researchers searching through case files, there is some evidence to suggest that it was not always acknowledged by social workers.'*
>
> *(WARD AND SKUSE 2001)*

Ward and Skuse point to placement plans given to carers at the time of placement which give no indication of mental health concerns which subsequently became apparent to carers:

'No information had been recorded in the Placement Plan at entry. However, the review form prior to Time 2 noted: "Very extreme and bizarre behaviour. Imagines something touching her and shouts 'Bloody keep off me'. Makes animal noises and body shakes uncontrollably." Will urinate publicly and in inappropriate places (living room, playing field). Obsession with death. Attempts to stab people. Very insecure. Needs constant reassurance.'

(IBID)

Despite such indications that some forms of mental distress might be going unnoticed, and hence under-recorded, the study by Ward and Skuse still found that a 'sizeable percentage' of the children on whom data was collected (over a third) had been seen by a mental health professional at some point in their lives.

The long-term impact of the LAC initiative remains to be assessed. But use of the records is clearly intended to provide a stimulus for social workers to obtain the necessary information, encourage collaboration between social workers, primary health care teams and other professionals, and facilitate the setting and monitoring of health goals.

'The early findings of the Looked After Children research indicate that using the system raises the awareness of social workers and carers about health issues, improves collaboration with primary health care teams and promotes a much more active approach to health and sex education.'

(JACKSON AND KILROE 1996)

Health records

As in England, other countries are also now recognising that continuity of care depends on good quality health records. At the Department du Nord in France, for instance, each looked after child's health records contain information such as medical history, family medical history, previous health assessments and treatment, and use of any specialist services, such as mental health services. The report of the young person's annual medical examination, which covers physical health, mental health, social presentation, behaviour and dental health, is also kept. Finally, a liaison note from the child's key worker sets out the actions to be taken to ensure the looked after child's health needs are met within the overall care plan. Parents continue to hold parental records, and it is their responsibility to complete these in relation to any health care the child might receive.

Researchers in Canada and California also referred to the importance of good child health records. Klee and others (1992) advocated use of a medical passport which would be given to all foster parents and contain a record of the child's health, including information such as any problems or special needs, actions taken, and recommendations for future treatment or intervention. This 'passport' would accompany a child to all health appointments and would remain with him or her through placements or an eventual return home. It would be developed in conjunction with the young person's care and treatment plan.

Keeping good records on young people from an early age was recognised by several respondents in the international survey as critical. Clare and Clare (2000) argued that, in Australia, a clearer recognition of a child's journey through care, would improve the health of looked after children. It would also lead to a better understanding of the factors that may have impacted on their health and health care. The Department du Nord in France reported on attempts to maintain longitudinal health records by providing an initial health assessment once children are admitted to care and carrying out subsequent assessments annually. A report from Canada recommended a health check within 24 hours of the child's admission to care, followed by a further complete assessment within one month of the child's placement. A report into California's child welfare services advocated a health check within 72 hours of a child or young person entering care to look for signs of abuse, neglect, communicable diseases, medical needs, pregnancy and suicidal tendencies. A comprehensive assessment should follow within 30 or 60 days.

Collaboration

Within England, despite the intentions of the LAC initiative to improve collaboration, there are clearly still problems in the effective sharing of information between the many individuals and agencies involved in looking after a young person in care. Mather and Batty found that:

> *'Medical and social assessments often occur in isolation. Medical advisers should discuss with their local social services departments how medical and social assessments can best be integrated locally and information sharing become more effective.'*
>
> *(MATHER AND BATTY 2000)*

Weaknesses in the collaborative process between health and social services were noted in the Social Services Inspectorate report *When Leaving Home is Also Leaving Care:*

> *'There was little evidence of joint work between health authorities and SSD's to develop strategies to overcome the disadvantages of young people leaving care or to link them into general programmes of health promotion.'*

The report also noted that social services departments had difficulties working with health authorities for this user group:

> *'Sometimes there was no "right person" in health to involve in planning, responsibilities for the relevant services could be with different purchasing managers within the health authority, and the services could be managed by different trusts or different directorates within a trust and health providers.'*
> *(DEPARTMENT OF HEALTH 1997B)*

Policy and practice context for promoting the health of looked after children

Standards and guidance

Many existing standards applied to children in care are concerned with illness rather than health, focusing on matters such as registration with a GP, medical assessments and developmental checks. However, several standards contain both explicit and implicit references to health promotion obligations for care providers.

The Children Act 1989 sets the statutory framework for young people in and leaving care. Volume 4 of the Act's Guidance and Regulations states that:

'Children in homes are particularly vulnerable as they frequently have not received continuity of health care because they have been subject to a sequence of moves, often within a fairly short time scale. Staff should play an active role in promoting all aspects of a child's health. Health care should include education about alcohol and other substance abuse, sexual matters, and HIV/AIDS and should not be restricted to treatment of illness and accidents.'

(DEPARTMENT OF HEALTH 1991)

In its report into promoting good practice within residential care, the Support Force for Children's Residential Care recommended that staff should take a planned and proactive approach to helping young people achieve healthier lifestyles. They should also engage with the local health promotion services to provide positive messages and accurate information for the young people in their care.

'... in the present day world, once children and young people begin to interact with a wider environment, they are exposed to influences which can be difficult to deal with, and which may be potentially dangerous. Good parenting in today's world therefore requires not only that children and young people are provided with the best opportunity for good health, but also that they are prepared for taking care of their own health and safety from a relatively early age.'

(SUPPORT FORCE FOR CHILDREN'S RESIDENTIAL CARE 1995)

An outcome in the Department of Health's document *Children's Homes – National Minimum Standards – Children's Homes Regulations* (DoH 2002a) states:

'Children live in a healthy environment and their health needs are identified and services are provided to meet them, and their good health is promoted.'

Standard 12.1, which supports the outcome, states:

'The physical, emotional and health needs of each child are identified and appropriate action is taken to secure the medical, dental and other health services needed to meet them. Children are provided with guidance, advice and support on health and personal care issues appropriate to the needs and wishes of each child.'

Each child should have a written health plan and records of illnesses, accidents and injuries; they should receive guidance and education concerning health promotion within specific areas, and each home should have a policy concerning health promotion. Children with specific health problems or a disability should also be provided with appropriate support and treatment and the needs of children from minority ethnic and cultural groups should be understood and addressed.

Other standards also help to promote the health and well-being of children. For instance, those relating to the provision of food and the opportunity to shop for and prepare their own meals (Standard 10); opportunities to take part in a range of appropriate leisure activities (Standard 15); and to live in well designed homes with sufficient space. Such factors are crucial to promoting the child's health and well-being and self-esteem, and will, if implemented, have a direct effect upon the child's emotional and mental health.

These requirements are mirrored in other standards for boarding schools (DoH 2002b), residential special schools (DoH 2002c), further education colleges (DoH 2002d) and fostering services (DoH 2002e) although they make allowances for these different settings and the different duties and responsibilities carried by the providers.

Other service standards and targets

Other service standards and targets which relate directly to health and well-being in care include the following:

- the Social Services Inspectorate's *Standards for Leaving Care* (DoH 1996) under Standard 9: Health and Personal Development and Standard 10: Employment/Education/Training.

- *Personal Social Services Performance Assessment Framework's* indicator C19, health assessments, dental checks and immunisation rates (Department of Health, Social Care Group 1999a)

- *Modernising Health and Social Services: National Priorities Guidance 1999 – 2000* (Department of Health 1999b) – the latter setting amongst other objectives, reductions in placement moves, improvement in educational qualifications, employment and training, increased numbers of looked after children having a comprehensive health assessment, and reducing the number of teenage pregnancies.

Policies and plans

Quality Protects

Recent legislative changes arguably represent an important sea change in the drive for improving standards directly affecting health and well-being. The regulations and guidance to the *Children (Leaving Care) Act 2000* specify that health considerations should form part of Pathway Planning (DoH 2001a).

The *Quality Protects* programme is another important advance, with its emphasis on specific objectives for improving health, placement stability, educational support and support for leaving care. *Quality Protects* has monitored the year-on-year performance of local authorities set against these key objectives.

Taken together, these should have a direct bearing upon health from a holistic perspective:

> *'Objective 4.0 – To ensure that children looked after gain maximum life chance benefits from educational opportunities, health care and social care ...*
>
> *Sub-objective 4.2 – To ensure that children looked after enjoy a standard of health and development as good as all children of the same age living in the same area ...*
>
> *Sub-objective 4.4 – To ensure that children from black and ethnic minority groups gain maximum life chance benefits from educational opportunities, health care and social care.'*
>
> *(DEPARTMENT OF HEALTH 1999B)*

The forthcoming National Service Framework for Children (NSF) will provide a framework for the strategic coordination of the broad spectrum of child health and social care services and policies across agencies.

National Overview Report of the Management Action Plans

The second *National Overview Report of the Management Action Plans*, submitted to the Department of Health by local authorities, already indicates improvements in some aspects of health care. For example increased percentages of looked after children who are up to date with their immunisations, visiting a dentist or who have had a comprehensive health assessment on entering care are recorded (Robbins 2000).

This may seem to demonstrate that indicators are focusing on measurable illness detection rather than the promotion of well-being. Yet the *overall* impact of the initiative, especially its objectives for improving placement stability, boosting educational achievement, and reducing the social isolation of care leavers, will certainly impact upon the self-esteem and well-being of young people in and leaving care. It also addresses some of the priorities set by young people themselves.

Signs of a shift to a more holistic approach to health care are explicit in the Department of Health's Guidance on *Promoting the Health of Looked After Children* (2002), which takes account of the wider determinants of health. It sets a context for partnership working involving statutory, voluntary and independent sectors, including education and leisure services, as well as health and social care, building on the views of children and young people.

> *'Effective corporate parenting should be supported by healthcare and health promotion policies which set out responsibilities at all levels of the organisation, and are developed in partnership with children, young people and their carers and other agencies.'*
>
> *(DEPARTMENT OF HEALTH 2002)*

There is a clear need for a holistic model of health, promoted by accessible services and infrastructure that empowers young people to take responsibility for their health and well-being. Evaluation of health education programmes, which do not address broader structural issues, offers ambivalent evidence of their value in reaching all sections of the community, especially those most at risk. It is essential therefore that health and well-being is promoted through political, organisational and individual attention to good practice.

The Department of Health Guidance on Promoting Health and Well Being (Department of Health 2002) for looked after children attaches great importance to this broad understanding of health and well-being, addressed through a child-centred model. This is identified in the well-being model (Buchanan and Hudson 2000, cited in DoH Guidance 2002, see Appendix 1).

> *'Good health goes beyond having access to health services. Improved health outcomes for looked after children require the focus for health and care planning to be on health promotion and attention to environmental factors as well as physical, emotional and mental health needs. Children and young people need to understand their right to good health and to be able to access services. They need the knowledge and skills to communicate and relate to others, and take responsibility for themselves.'*
>
> *(DEPARTMENT OF HEALTH, 2002)*

The current socio-political climate

The current health and social policy agenda of the Government includes a number of initiatives intended to reduce social exclusion and its costly consequences for society at large. The needs of looked after children are specifically targeted within several such initiatives. Arguably, this presents a unique opportunity to improve the health and life chances of looked after children. Since the Children's Safeguards Review (Utting 1997), the Ministerial Task Force's response (1998), and the inception of the Quality Protects programme, there has been an increasing focus on tackling the longstanding neglect of health and other interrelated issues for looked after children.

'The health needs of looked after children seem to the Review to be fundamental to keeping them safe. The Department of Health should facilitate the action needed by local and health authorities to identify and meet the health needs of looked after children.'

(UTTING 1997)

In 1997, the SSI identified a number of structural and management weaknesses in how departments were addressing young people's health. This included 'little evidence of joint work between health authorities and SSDs to develop strategies to overcome the disadvantage of young people leaving care or to link them into general programmes of health promotion.' (Department of Health 1997b)

Wyler (2000) argues we must take advantage of this favourable socio-political context to achieve real improvements in the health prospects of children in and leaving care:

'Over the last two years, the desire to improve services for young people in care and those leaving care has been high on the central and local government policy agenda. The Quality Protects programme, the Children (Leaving Care) Bill, and the Beacon Programme, are all serious attempts to raise standards and promote good practice. Health issues are beginning to receive more attention. There is therefore a more positive climate for innovation and improvement.'

(WYLER 2000)

Key policy issues from the literature and practice

Moving away from a disease model

Much of the literature concerned with the health of looked after children and young people relates to indices or accounts of ill health (Mather 2000b). The focus is upon identifying and reducing illness through medical interventions such as statutory health examinations, inoculations, and recording measures of the absence of 'illness'. The so-called 'medical' or 'disease' models of health have preoccupied much of the time and attention given to health by professionals working with children in care. Several writers have commented on the apparent preoccupation of literature and guidance with the annual statutory medical examinations, despite the evidence of poor take-up, consumer resentment, and indications that recommendations arising from the examinations are rarely acted upon (Mather and Batty 2000, Polnay 2000). Mather and Batty (2000) point out 'no other group of children in the population is subject to this statutory requirement', which is much resented by young people themselves:

> *'Having to take your clothes off for a strange doctor, when you don't feel ill is yet one more abuse of the system.'*
>
> *(MATHER AND OTHERS 1997 AS CITED IN MATHER AND BATTY 2000)*

The feeling that the system is 'processing' the young people without achieving the desired result of improved health and care, requires a radical reassessment of health care and health promotion – one which listens to and acts upon the views and experience of young people themselves:

> *'Why should a system with so many legal safeguards, and to which a large amount of health service resources are devoted, produce such an unsatisfactory situation, both for the consumers of the service, and for doctors and social workers? ...*
>
> *A radically new approach is needed for the future in the health provision for these children. This approach should concentrate on holistic health care with an emphasis on health rather than illness.'*
>
> *(MATHER AND BATTY 2000)*

The findings of Saunders and Broad's study, confirmed by an earlier Save the Children report (West 1995) which was researched by young careleavers, have important implications for those seeking to improve the health of looked after children:

> '... for the young careleavers interviewed, health was not just, or even primarily, about eating the right things, not smoking or drinking and having access to primary health care services. It was about being a paid up member of society, being in a position to make positive health choices, having good things going on in their lives and hope for the future, a secure home, good social relationships and happier care experiences.'
>
> *(SAUNDERS AND BROAD 1997)*

Towards holistic health and well-being

Holistic health

A holistic model of health is concerned with far more than an absence of illness:

> 'A state of complete physical, mental and social well being and not merely the absence of disease or infirmity.'
>
> *(WHO 1946)*

This definition clearly sets the boundaries of health far wider than the purely medical model. The definition is 'holistic' in that it considers all aspects of a person's life and experience.

Seedhouse (1986) favours a person-centred concept of health as a foundation for achievement, qualified by the many factors affecting the opportunity for its realisation. The model is one, which is holistic, acknowledging the many varied factors, which affect an individual. Health is a base from which to develop, enabling people to do or choose to do as many things as possible to achieve their potential.

'What health means to me?'

- running and playing
- being with my friends
- on my bike and exercise
- eating food, fruit
- sleeping at night and good dreams

13-YEAR-OLD BOY

PARTICIPATING IN NATIONAL CHILDREN'S BUREAU HEALTH PROJECT (LEWIS 1999)

Seedhouse's definition, relates to the individual's needs, and is exemplified above. When used alongside the World Health Organisation (WHO) definition, it is an aspirational one, which seems to correspond more closely with the views of young people themselves when asked to say what health means to them (Saunders and Broad 1997, Lewis 1999, Wyler 2000)

The UN Convention on the Rights of the Child has been adopted by national governments and its elements underpin the health and well-being of all children, explicitly stated by Article 24 which identifies the child's right to the best health possible and to medical care. The right to safety and protection, appropriate care and adequate living standards, access to education, leisure and cultural activities and freedom of expression, are some of the provisions that contribute to the holistic health and well-being of all children.

Article 12 states that children should have a say in decisions that affect their lives. In Saunders and Broad (1997) an account is given of how a group of young people have developed their own model of holistic health in consultation with researchers. This model provides their understanding of whole health.

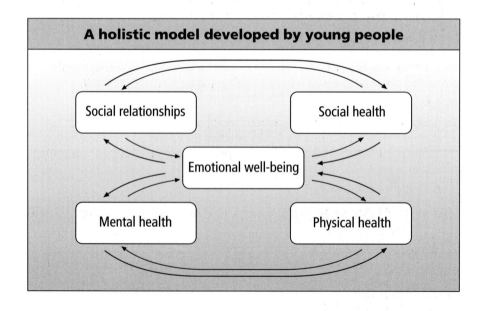

A holistic model developed by young people

Social relationships

Social health

Emotional well-being

Mental health

Physical health

Saunders and Broad, the researchers, explain that the model is based on the premise that there is no such thing as being '100 per cent healthy' and that health is a relative concept which relates to a number of life contexts:

> 'The model has two dimensions, the personal and the social, each having a number of key elements. In the personal dimension the main aspects relating to health are mental, physical and emotional states, whilst in the social dimension they are relationships and practical issues, for example employment and housing. No one dimension or aspect is more important than any other. All interrelate and changes, whether positive or negative, in any one aspect will in turn influence the others. Within this model good health is a very individual matter and is largely a result of making choices and finding a positive balance across these dimensions and elements.'
>
> (SAUNDERS AND BROAD 1997)

This model demonstrates that health promotion must address the broad determinants of health through policy, empowerment and education.

Frameworks for promoting health and well-being

The first World Health Organisation International Conference on Health Promotion, held in 1986, which led to the Ottawa Charter (WHO 1987), developed a framework for the delivery of health promotion programmes. Five principle areas for health promotion action were identified:

- building healthy public policies;
- creating supportive environments;
- strengthening community action;
- developing personal skills;
- reorientating health services.

Three methodologies were also identified through which people could begin to take control of their own health:

- mediation;
- enablement;
- advocacy.

These actions and methodologies provide a basic framework for the delivery of health promotion programmes. All populations are entitled to minimum standards of health, and these cannot be achieved at the expense of one individual for another

(MacDonald 1993).

In her training pack for residential social workers and foster carers, Lewis (1999) offers the following definition of health promotion:

> *'[It] can be defined as the process of enabling people to increase control over the determinants of health and thereby improve their health. It acknowledges the interdependent roles of health education, health protection, prevention and community participation in creating health literacy, personal health skills and supportive environments for health. For younger children, the focus is on giving them information about how to look after their health and the factors which affect their health, helping them to develop the skills they need to protect their health as they grow and mature. For older children and young people, who have developed the skills and ability to reason and make choices with respect to their longer term future, it is essentially about empowerment – increasing autonomy, independence and self-determination.'*
>
> *(LEWIS 1999)*

Various models of health promotion exist to help clarify the purpose of intervention. A commonly used model by Tannahill (1994) identifies three elements of health promotion as health education, health protection and the prevention of ill health, and identifies their interrelations. Another model identifies a simple connection between healthy public policy and health education (Tones and others 1990, see Appendix 3).

These models indicate the importance of empowering children and young people to take control of their well-being, supported through the policy, organisation and cultural changes that are necessary to provide them with a healthy, caring environment.

In her chapter on promoting well-being (in Buchanan and Hudson 2000) Sarah Stewart Brown shows how healthy public policy, and the social well-being in communities and workplaces affects the well-being of children and their parents and carers. This model is cited in the Health Guidance (DoH 2002).

Involving young people in the development and delivery of services

While it is difficult to measure the effectiveness of some health policy interventions, it is plausible to argue that listening and responding to young people's priorities when framing health policies will increase the acceptability and therefore take-up of services.

Children's participation is a major strand of work undertaken within the Quality Protects Initiative. It is also being forwarded through other national strategies including the National Service Framework for Children, and Children and Young People's Unit work on Core Principles for Children and Young People's Participation in Government.

> 'We do not know enough about the effectiveness in terms of outcomes of involving children and young people in agenda setting, however, evidence from other areas of healthcare, in particular childbirth, suggests that a user-driven agenda makes for services which are more accessible and acceptable.'
>
> (ROBERTS 2000)

The international review also highlights awareness in other countries of involving young people more in their own health care. A report from Canada suggested that adolescents should be provided with preventative health services and information on subjects such as sexuality, reproduction, substance misuse and smoking (Simms 1991 *mentioned in* Kudfeldt and others 2000). They should also be given the opportunity to see a doctor of their own choosing and to take part in their assessment and treatment (Mather and others *mentioned in* Kudfeldt and others 2000).

To be successful, health improvement programmes need more than the reluctant consent of the young person, they require their active participation and empowerment as the primary custodians of their own health. Many parents will confirm how difficult it can be to interest their children in long-term health matters, and the corporate parent faces even more difficulty in this respect.

> '... health promotion (or health education) is often viewed as merely the provision of information to individuals to persuade them to live healthier lifestyles. Most people working in the field however accept that while information giving is an important element, developing structures to enable people to have healthier lives is as important, if not more so ... where health promotion work is to be undertaken directly with the population in question, the aim is not necessarily to give directives about health, but also help individuals or groups to develop skills to prepare them for decisions that can influence health, for example how to resist peer pressure, or how to negotiate safer sex.'
>
> (MCGUIRE AND CORLYON 1997)

Young people's views on improving services

Wyler (2000), in his report on the health needs of young people leaving care, identified key issues for services, based on comments from young people. These include:

- Access to health care should be improved, both before and after leaving care. Young people should have regular health checks and receive advice about drugs, alcohol, sex and contraception, and their individual health needs.

  'The preparation for leaving care should involve visits to medical practitioners and definitely be conducted on an individual basis. The preparation process should cover how to register with practit oners, use of hospitals, payment of treatment, food and cooking (including training), drugs (including alcohol and smoking), sex and contraception, and some basic heath education on how to look after yourself ... preparation work should be done by doctors and nurses, perhaps in connection with social workers and running workshops.'

- Training on living independently should be available. It should include practical and life skills such as cooking and budgeting.

- Young people should be encouraged to make their own decisions, and their views should be listened to.

  'Young people should be encouraged and supported to make their own decisions between 16 and 18 years of age. Young people should be consulted more, and have their views heard and acted upon at reviews and elsewhere.'

  'Counselling should be offered both while preparing to leave and after leaving care.'

  'There should be a fast track system for young people leaving care to access benefits. Extra funding is needed to access dentists, opticians, leisure facilities, education and training.'

- The services provided should meet the needs of the young people, not the needs of those providing help. Young people should be treated as individuals and staff need to be compassionate, realistic, honest, understanding and interested.

  'Access to services should be made easier and less stigmatising (the term mental health services is threatening and discouraging); better referral systems, especially from doctors to counsellors.'

  'Professionals should treat young people as individuals, and work with them in seeking solutions, not telling them what to do.'

Role and status of child care workers

The social pedagogue

One approach used in some European countries to develop a more young person-centred model is the training of residential child care workers as social pedagogues. The role of the social pedagogue is to 'bring up' the child in all areas of life rather than just to respond to identified need in specific areas.

Kornbeck (2000) describes pedagogy as being:

> '... more concerned with preventative intervention and is much more linked to philosophy and psychology, than to sociology and social work.'

Other authors have described how:

> 'Social pedagogy draws on ideas of social reform, renewing society through the skill of developing a person's inherent potential.'
>
> *(CANNAN, BERRY AND LYONS 1992 MENTIONED IN KUFELDT AND OTHERS 2000)*

> 'Social pedagogues use preventative, developmental, and educative forms of intervention with communities of users (not just children), and deliver ideas of developmental support through more informal means than classroom education.'
>
> *(HIGHAM 2001)*

Pat Petrie at the Thomas Coram Research Unit looked at the role of the pedagogue in Denmark, Flanders, Netherlands and Germany. She has consulted with professionals in education and social welfare, and carried out focus groups with young people. She stresses that fundamental to social pedagogy is the act of listening to the child, reflecting and then responding. The pedagogue and the child work together on activities such as drama, music and art, and form a mutual bond. The aim is that the child's self-esteem will develop through the relationship between the adult and child, and that the child's physical and psychosocial health needs are addressed within an everyday setting. This type of holistic approach, Petrie suggests, is key to meeting the health needs of looked after children.

There is considerable variation across Europe both in terms of the training necessary to become a qualified social pedagogue (about four years on average), and the proportion working with looked after children who are likely to be trained (Petrie 2001). State residential settings mostly employ pedagogues although teachers, psychologists, social workers and counsellors also have a role and will have received training in pedagogic principles.

Status of child care workers

The other important difference between residential child care workers in England and in many other countries is their status. Traditionally, residential child care workers outside England have had higher status and levels of training. This factor is likely to have a considerable impact on the capacity of residential staff to meet the complex needs of young people who are looked after, including their health needs.

Joined up services

Shifting the Balance of Power (DoH 2001b) has created major structural changes in the configuration of health services from area and regional health authorities to Strategic Health Authorities with the majority of health care provided through Primary Care Trusts. There will be strengthening of relationships both within local authorities and across government, and the adoption of a public health approach to address inequalities and the wider health determinants. Children and young people will need to be a significant priority for these emerging and developing structures and services if needs are to be adequately noted and resourced. The National Service Framework for Children, with its overview of all children's services will be an essential vehicle for this.

It is now widely accepted that multi-agency partnerships are essential in tackling health improvement objectives. An issue of NCB's *Children Now* carried an account of a partnership between Southend-on-Sea's Social Services and the South Essex Health Authority. Its purpose was to set up a multi-agency/multidisciplinary *Health of Children Looked After Forum*. It is intended that this would act as a focus for health improvement, become a mechanism for assessing the mental health needs and emotional well-being of looked after children, and for reviewing the uptake of routine immunisations and the role of annual health assessments. Closer joint working between health and social services is seen as one of the major gains of the collaboration and *'a number of joint health promotion initiatives have been developed as a result,* (Atherton and Munday 2000).

The *Quality Protects Newsletter* for December 2000 contains another example of a social service/health partnership, in Southampton and described as 'a dedicated, centralised health service for looked after children'. Benefits claimed are priority access to mental health services and dental care, regular liaison with a psychologist, a database of key health information for looked after children and health care planning in 'language understandable to all'. Acknowledging that 'routine medicals' for children and young people are archaic and desperately in need of revision, Dr Cathy Hill, the project leader, states that:

'If we want to address the real health problems of these children we must deliver services that are appropriate to their needs, not those of the professionals.'

(HILL 2000)

The service has concentrated on the needs of teenage groups, who are least likely to attend health assessments but are more vulnerable to health risk behaviours such as drug abuse or unsafe sex. The service has worked to provide advice and health services in a setting and format which is attractive and relevant to young people – offering health assessments and information at a local leisure centre:

'We have moved on from "You will come for a medical" – which they don't come to – to an environment, complete with pop videos in the waiting area, which is attractive to them. It's early days but so far it seems to be a good way of hooking them into services.'

(IBID)

In line with present-day thinking in Britain, most countries taking part in the international review indicated the importance of interagency working. It was generally felt that young people's health needs are best met if services work together to this end. The Department du Nord in France, for instance, has a policy of working with a range of health professionals to help develop each child's care plan.

A view from Canada (Klee and others 1992 *cited in* Kufeldt and others 2000) recommended that policies for looked after children's health services should be written and shared with involved agencies *and* all associated professions. Multidisciplinary teams were advocated (Simms 1991 *mentioned in* Kufeldt and others 2000) for making decisions about children, and the benefits of physicians acting as advisors to social workers when addressing children's health needs and suitable placements were maintained. Using case managers to share responsibility for coordinating children's health care was also recommended (Berkowitz and others, mentioned in Kufeldt and others 2000).

The health camps in New Zealand, Australia and Munich (see page 35) also advocated the integration of health services for young people who attended.

Examples of good practice

'Systematic collection of data about young care leavers, and comparisons over time, in order to chart an individual's personal progress, or to assess the impact of services, is extremely weak.'

(WYLER 2000)

There is a serious dearth of literature on what can be 'proved' to work in this area of practice. Not only has the health of looked after children been a neglected area of practice until recently, but there are difficulties in terms of what can be measured, which outcome can be linked to which intervention, and the interacting, cumulative and variable nature of the factors which result in health or ill health. Hence, many initiatives are not as yet rigorously tested and little work has been done on assessing their impact on behaviour.

One exception cited by Wyler is the Signpost project in Wakefield, which carries out annual surveys of the children with whom they work, including users who represent 92 per cent of the local care population. Their surveys indicate that the number of teenage pregnancies has declined sharply over a three-year period from 14 to five, and they suggest that this reduction results primarily from the personal development programmes which they offer and many other positive initiatives are cited.

Developed on a holistic model, they offer practical help and support to young people as well as involving them in the running and management of services. Kensington and Chelsea Social Services has established a multidisciplinary steering group on the mental health of children in need. It has also set up a drop-in service – 'A Place to Talk' – for young people in and leaving care, which is staffed by an experienced multidisciplinary team including a social worker, a child psychotherapist, a pupil referral unit manager and a health information project manager. The steering group is looking to develop the involvement of young people in promoting and publicising the service.

In Stockport, the youth service and health authority have jointly established a 'Central Youth' shopfront service where the 'Head to Head' project provides counselling services and a healthy lifestyles programme. The service has links to the Stockport Health Improvement Programme, helping young people register with a GP and arranging referrals to other appropriate health promotion agencies.

The 'Take Control, Take Care' young people's health project in Lewisham, supported by the Social Services Leaving and Aftercare Team, First Key, The Children's Society and Lewisham Health Action Zone, is training young people to carry out a health audit. Barnardo's Leaving Care Service in Manchester has produced a health pack with the help of young people and is looking to develop work on teenage pregnancy with the local hospital and Health Action Zone.

In the international review, New Zealand, Australia, and Munich provided details of health camps organised to meet the special needs of children and young people. Although these tended to focus on young people with specific medical conditions, they could in principle be extended to looked after young people. The camps take a holistic approach to children's health and aim to develop a child's self-esteem, confidence and independence. They offer a secure and supportive environment for children in which access to medical services and highly trained staff are provided. In New Zealand, health camps funded by the government are offered to children all year round to meet specific needs, including social and life skills, asthma management, diabetes management, skin care and enuresis. Similar initiatives are available in England but it may be that practice in this country could benefit from a closer examination of how such camps operate elsewhere.

The creation of a safe environment is particularly important for children in residential settings. Being able to both evaluate how safe the environment is and to engage children in making it safe are key in meeting these needs. One tool that enables both professional evaluation and children's participation is a checklist for safe environments (Varnava 1999). It raises awareness and establishes commitment from schools to promote nonviolence within schools and the wider community.

Much health supporting and enabling work in England is associated with local authority leaving care initiatives designed to help young people make successful transitions to independence. For example, four local authorities, Kensington and Chelsea, Suffolk, Wakefield and Westminster, have been selected as 'beacon' authorities for their work with careleavers. (Wyler 2000). A multi-agency Health Needs Forum has been established in Surrey to address the health needs of young people leaving care, to develop a strategy for a new mental health service and to examine how to measure health outcomes.

The *Quality Protects* website contains a 'good practice' database which includes projects from across the country which are undertaking work geared to improving the health of looked after children. These cover areas of concern such as drug misuse, teenage pregnancy, sexual health, mental health, personal relationships and loneliness, and support services to children with disabilities. However the introductory 'page' to the database states that:

'The Department of Health is not able to evaluate any of the examples given, entries reflect local circumstance and what works well in one area may not in another ... there are no selection criteria ...'

(HTTP://WWW.DOH.GOV.UK/QUALITYPROTECTS/QP_DATABASE/INDEX.HTM)

The examples given therefore are essentially self-assessed as to their value and merit as 'good practice' and although useful for stimulating discussion tell us little as to what works best in improving health outcomes.

However, despite such examples of good practice detailed above, and the *'positive climate for innovation and improvement'*, the pattern of work being undertaken across the country is still patchy. A study of 1999 – 2000 Health Improvement Plans carried out by the NSPCC found that the issue of looked after children and health ranked seventh in the 'Top Ten' most commonly addressed health issues and the key focus of the work proposed was centred around the development of individual health assessments, records and plans (Brunt 1999). Medicine and a medical model of health and health promotion is one strand of holistic health. Further work is required to improve the holistic health of young people, addressing structuralist and educational issues, thus empowering young people to have greater control over their health and well-being.

Current developments

National Service Framework for Children

The National Service Framework (NSF) for Children is currently being developed to determine the future delivery of children's health services. It will set standards for health and social care services for all children, including those who are looked after. It is essential therefore that the work of the National Healthy Care Standard is placed within this planning and delivery framework and is supported by the NSF.

National Healthy Care Standard and National Healthy School Standard

The National Healthy Care Standard will promote a healthy care environment based on an understanding that partnerships between agencies, and the participation of young people and those who are responsible for their care, is essential for success. It will provide a local structure, mirrored nationally, including social care, health and education working together to develop a programme in which the outcomes of the NHCS can be carried out. These are that children and young people who are looked after will:

- live in an environment that promotes health and well-being, within the wider community;
- experience a genuinely caring, consistent, stable and secure relationship with at least one committed, trained, experienced and supported carer;
- be given opportunities to develop personally and socially to take responsibility for their health and well-being now and in the future;
- receive excellent quality health care assessments, treatment and support.

These outcomes will be demonstrated through a nationally accredited scheme, which supports effective policy, practice and partnership working, and involves children and young people's participation through the process.

The development of the NHCS can draw on, and learn from, the clear guidance already in place with the National Healthy School Standard (NHSS):

'Social services departments are experiencing some difficulties in maintaining a focus on improving health outcomes for the children in their care. There might be useful parallels to be drawn with promoting health in schools, The National Healthy School Standard (NHSS), is now established in every local authority funded locally by the LEA and Health Authority/Trust, and nationally by the DfEE and Department of Health. The NHSS offers schools an achievable model of

health improvement which both raises pupils' academic achievement and provides support for personal, social and health education.'

(LEWIS 2000)

The concept of the Health Promoting School was first developed in the early 1980s by the World Health Organisation. It was intended to be:

'... a means of encouraging a holistic, whole school approach to personal and community health within the school setting ... the original concept has been translated into practice in many countries across Europe. There has been a steady growth of healthy schools schemes and projects, including local awards, in the UK over recent years.'

(RIVERS AND OTHERS 1999)

The *NHSS Guidance* outlines the purpose of the healthy schools programmes, which are based in education and health partnerships, as being to provide support to schools in becoming healthier places for staff and pupils to work and learn and to improve education standards. Additionally the NHSS aims to promote inclusion through addressing social and health inequalities. The partnerships offer guidance and support on a range of health related topics and activities undertaken in different contexts – for example Personal, Social and Health Education and Citizenship education – and in partnership with other agencies. All this is geared towards producing a:

'... supportive whole school practice ... more likely to have a greater impact on pupils' health, learning opportunities, experience and indeed, their achievements.'

(DFEE 1999)

The NHSS offers support to local programme coordinators and provides an accreditation process for education and health partnerships, intended to give them consistency, credibility and status, and thereby increase the effectiveness of their work with schools.

Schools which can meet the criteria for participation, providing evidence to demonstrate the achievement of the national quality standards can achieve recognition as a 'healthy school' and use the Healthy Schools' logo. Becoming a 'healthy school' is seen as a developmental process which will be ongoing – maintaining progress and setting new targets.

'[The] National Healthy School Standard is aimed principally at whole school improvement, but as it is instrumental in developing agency co-ordination and improved access to health advice for young people, the initiative will form part of overall planning for children's services ... a key aspect of the Standard is partnership working between LEA's and Health Authorities (to form Education and Health Partnerships), with input from relevant departments and agencies such as Social Services, Drug Action Teams, Police and Primary Care Groups or Trusts, to help achieve health improvement. There are eight themes underlying the Standard including emotional health and well-being, education about drugs, alcohol, bullying, and tobacco. Accreditation requires that schools achieve a national standard with respect to equity, pupils having a voice, partnership with parents, carers and the local community.'

(DEPARTMENT OF HEALTH 2000B)

The NHSS addresses health through partnerships between education and health as well as Primary Care Trusts and Social Services departments and youth work agencies. It involves staff and young people at both strategic and operational levels. NHCS is being developed in parallel with this process. It will take into account the whole context and culture of a child or young person in local authority care and preparing for life outside of care.

Conclusion

An important conclusion to the literature reviewed both nationally and internationally is that the health of the looked after children should be considered holistically; the term health and well-being is used to clarify this. Agencies need to work together to establish systems that support carers and young people. NHSS provides a model of interagency working relevant to promoting health and well-being. Staff in agencies working with young people in care need information, training and support to equip them with skills, knowledge and values that contribute to a healthy care environment. It is the coordinated development of policies, partnerships and improved practice that will empower young people to take control of their health and well-being, supported within a healthy care environment as required by the Department of Health Guidance on promoting health of looked after children delivered through the National Healthy Care Standard.

Arguably, the training, orientation and status of child care workers are key areas to address if services are to improve. While the European social pedagogue model may not be easily transported into the care setting, serious consideration should be given to how it might be adapted and translated into the English child care role across a number of sectors. The emphasis on taking the 'whole child' into account is important, and addresses the need to take a holistic perspective on a young person's life. The emphasis on the development of a relationship between child and carer is also likely to be critical. This will lead to a better understanding of the young person's needs and ideas on how these might be met, is likely to encourage compliance with any strategies identified, and to contribute more generally to enhanced self-esteem and emotional well-being.

Training for pedagogues includes the study of theory of relevant methods (such as group work skills), practice placements and frequently a range of arts, crafts, music, drama and practical skills like gardening, that staff will be able to use in their work with young people. More generally, it is worth rethinking the issue of status within the profession and asking whether, on the whole, higher status workers might be expected to provide higher quality services.

Another key challenge borne out by both reviews is the need for continuity and consistency in health care, and the positive impact this can have on mental and emotional well-being. This follows in many ways from the concept of the relationship with the pedagogue highlighted above, and is related to the aspects of joined up services and good quality health records that have also been described. The notion of a health 'passport', which is not unknown in England, may also be valuable.

The NHCS promotes a model for changing the culture within the public care system, which has too often appeared to accept, and even compound, the poor health outcomes for many 'looked after' young people. It will provide a holistic framework for tackling health issues and offer support mechanisms and structures for ongoing improvement and development – as such its viability and potential for the care sector is promising. Further work will be needed to identify and address the factors that impact on the health and well-being of looked after children. The NHCS will provide this opportunity by helping to identify, monitor and evaluate good practice and to support the development of work to acknowledge and address the identified gaps.

Finally, a more focused international inquiry into specific areas of health care, including those outlined in this report, may be helpful in developing the NHCS. This needs to be carried out in a detailed and systematic manner, paying attention to issues of sustainability, quality and effectiveness on the one hand, and young people's participation and satisfaction on the other. It is only with evidence-based knowledge of provision, which includes appropriate comparative data and evaluation, that we can have any real clues to the way forward.

The development and implementation of NHCS is founded on a belief that all children are entitled to excellent, consistant care and health care, and a care environment that will equip them with the knowledge, skills and values for life now and in the future. This public health approach to addressing the inequalities of children's health and well-being will be enabled through placing the NHCS as a key deliverable in the National Service Framework for Children.

Appendix 1

THE WELL-BEING MODEL OF HEALTH (REPRODUCED FROM STEWART-BROWN, S. PARENTING, SCHOOLING AND CHILDREN'S BEHAVIOUR IN BUCHANAN AND HUDSON 2002)

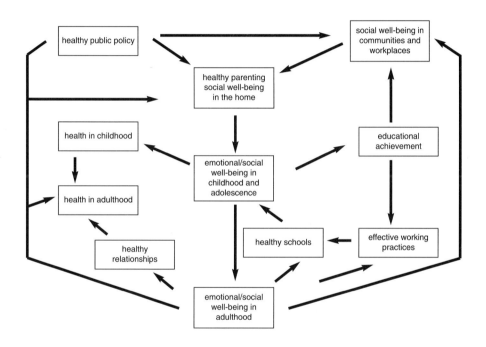

Appendix 2

WARD, H AND SKUSE, T (2001) *LOOKING AFTER CHILDREN: USING DATA AS MANAGEMENT INFORMATION. REPORT FROM THE FIRST YEAR OF DATA COLLECTION.*

TABLE 8: EVIDENCE OF VULNERABILITY

	Frequency	% (groups not discrete)
Health	134	54
Education	102	41
Identity	57	23
Family and Social Relationships	183	74
Social Presentation	60	24
Emotional and Behavioural Development	126	51
Self Care Skills	47	19

TABLE 9: ONGOING HEALTH CONDITIONS FOR TOTAL SAMPLE

Health condition	Valid percentage (groups not discrete)
Asthma	17.8
Coeliac disease	0.5
Epilepsy	8.5
Hayfever	1.9
Thalassaemia	0.5
Hearing impairment	8.9
Learning disability	18.3
Cerebral palsy	4.2
Cystic fibrosis	0.5
Eczema	9.3
Glue ear	2.8
Visual impairment	9.3
Physical disability or mobility problems	8.0
Other chronic condition requiring outpatient appointments	19.5

TABLE 10: INCIDENCE OF LEARNING DISABILITY BY LOCAL AUTHORITY

Local Authority	Percentage of children with learning disabilities
Authority A	50
Authority B	23.8
Authority C	17.2
Authority D	77.8
Authority E	6.3
Authority F	12.7

TABLE 11: TYPE AND PREVALENCE OF BEHAVIOUR PROBLEMS (119 CHILDREN)

Problem behaviour	Frequency	Percentage noted at 1.4.98 (not discreet)
Conduct disorder (not related to ongoing health condition)	78	33.1
Conduct disorder (related to ongoing health condition)	4	1.7
Conduct disorder (unclear if related to health)	1	0.4
Self harming behaviour	19	8.1
Inappropriate sexual behaviour	19	8.1
Relationship problems	18	7.6
Anxiety	14	5.9
Bedwetting (related to anxiety)	14	5.9
Bedwetting (related to health)	4	1.6
Concentration problems	7	3.0
Other Problem	8	3.4

Appendix 3

THE CONTRIBUTION OF EDUCATION TO HEALTH PROMOTION.
ADAPTED FROM TONES, CITED IN NAIDOO AND WILLIS, 1994.

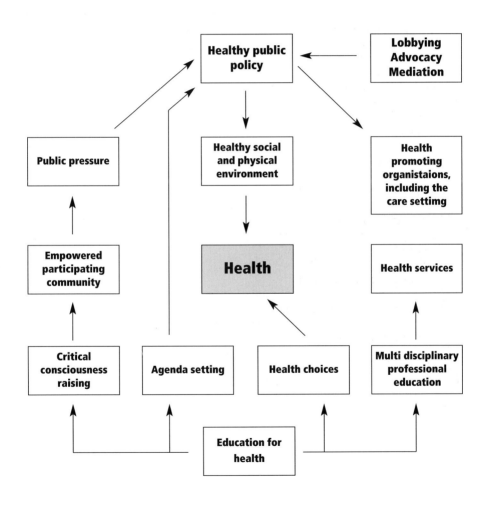

References

Acheson, D (1998) *Independent Inquiry into Inequalities in Health*. Stationery Office

Aggleton, P, Hurry, J and Warwick, I (2000) *Young People and Mental Health*. Wiley

Arcelus, J, Bellerby, T and Vostanis, P (1999) A mental health service for young people in the care of the local authority, *Clinical Child Psychology and Psychiatry*, 4, 2, 233-245

Atherton, A and Munday, C (2000) Tackling the health agenda for looked after children: lessons from Southend on Sea, *Children Now*, 6 (Autumn), 6-7

Bamford, F and Wolkind, SN (1988) *The Physical and Mental Health of Children in Care: Research needs*. ESRC

Barth, RP and Blackwell, DL (1998) Death rates among California's foster care and former foster care populations, *Child and Youth Service Review*, 20, 7, 577-604

Berkowitz and others (1992) *in* Kufeldt, K and others (2000) *Looking After Children in Canada*. University of New Brunswick

Biehal, N and others (1995) *Moving On: Young people and leaving care schemes*. Barnardo's

Biehal, N and others (1992) *Prepared for Living? A survey of young people leaving the care of three local authorities*. National Children's Bureau

Bignall, T and Butt J (2000) *Between Ambition and Achievement: Young black disabled people's views and experiences of independence and independent living*. Policy Press

Brodie, I, Berridge, D and Beckett, W (1997) The health of children looked after by local authorities, *British Journal of Nursing*, 6, 386-390

Brunt, S (1999) *Improving Children's Health: A survey of 1999-2000 health improvement programmes*. NSPCC

Buchanan, A (1999) Are care leavers significantly dissatisfied and depressed in adult life? *Adoption and Fostering*, 23, 4, 35-40

Buchanan, A and Hudson, B eds. (2000) *Promoting Children's Emotional Well-being*. Oxford University Press

Butler, I and Payne, H (1997) The health of children looked after by the local authority, *Adoption and Fostering*, 21, 2 28-35

Cain and Barth (1990) in Kufeldt and others (2000) *Looking After Children in Canada*. University of New Brunswick

Cannan, C, Berry, L and Lyons, K (1992) *Social Work and Europe*. BASW/Macmillan Press

Clare, B (2001) Managing the care journey: Meeting the health care needs of children in out-of-home care. *Children Australia* 26, 1, 27 -33

Corlyon, J and McGuire, C (1997) *Young Parents in Public Care: Pregnancy and parenthood among young people looked after by local authorities.* National Children's Bureau

Department for Education and Employment (1999) *Healthy Schools: National Healthy School Standard Guidance.* DfEE

Department of Health (2002) *Promoting Health for Looked After Children.* DoH

Department of Health (2002a) *Children's Homes: National minimum standards. Children's homes regulations.* Stationery Office

Department of Health (2002b) *Boarding Schools: National minimum standards. Inspection regulations.* Stationery Office

Department of Health (2002c) *Residential Special Schools: National minimum standards. Inspection regulations.* Stationery Office

Department of Health (2002d) *Accommodation of Students Under Eighteen by Further Education Colleges: National minimum standards. Inspection regulations.* Stationery Office

Department of Health (2002e) *Fostering Services: National minimum standards. Fostering services regulations.* Stationery Office

Department of Health (2001a) *Children (Leaving Care) Act: Draft regulations and guidance.* DoH

Department of Health (2001b) *Shifting the Balance of Power.* DoH

Department of Health (2000) *Promoting Health for Looked After Children. A guide to healthcare planning, assessment and monitoring. Consultation document.* DoH

Department of Health. Social Care Group. Government Statistical Service (1999a) *Social Services Performance in 1998-99. The Personal Social Services Performance Assessment Framework.* DoH

Department of Health (1999b) *Modernising Health and Social Services: National priorities guidance 1999/00-2001/02.* (HSC 1999/126: LAC (99)22)

Department of Health (1999c) *The Government's Objectives for Children's Social Services.* DoH

Department of Health (1997a) *Substance Misuse and Young People: the social services response. A Social Services Inspectorate study of young people looked after by local authorities.* DoH

Department of Health (1997b) *When Leaving Home is also Leaving Care: an inspection of services for young people leaving care.* DoH

Department of Health (1996) *SSI Standards in Leaving Care.* DoH

Department of Health (1995) *Looking After Children: Good parenting, good outcomes. Training resources pack.* HMSO

Department of Health (1994) *Standards for Residential Child Care Services.* DoH

Department of Health (1991) *The Children Act 1989 Guidance and Regulations. Volume 4 Residential Care.* Stationery Office

Dimigen, G and others (1999) Psychiatric disorder among children at time of entering local authority care: questionnaire survey, *British Medical Journal*, 319, 675

Garland, AF and Besinger, RA (1997) Racial/ethnic differences in court referred pathways to mental health services for children in foster care, *Children and Youth Services Review*, 19, 8, 651- 666

Higham, P (2001) Changing practice and an emerging social pedagogue paradigm in England, *Social Work in Europe*, 8, 1, 21-29

Hill, C (2000) Dedicated to young people's health, *Quality Protects Newsletter*, 6 (December), 18-19

House of Commons. Health Committee (1998) *Children Looked After by Local Authorities. Second Report. Volume 1: Report and proceedings of the committee.* Stationery Office

Jackson, S and Kilroe, S eds. (1996) *Looking After Children: Good parenting, good outcomes. Reader.* HMSO

Kahan, B (1989) *Child Care Research, Policy and Practice.* Hodder and Stoughton

Karpilow, K, Burden, L and Carbaugh, L (1998) *Health Services for Children in Foster Care.* Institute for Research on Women and Families: California

Klee and others (1992) *mentioned in* Kufeldt, K and others (2000) *Looking After Children in Canada.* University of New Brunswick

Kornbeck, J (2000) Social work versus social pedagogy, *Professional Social Work*, Nov 2000, 12-13

Kufeldt, K and others (2000) *Looking After Children in Canada.* University of New Brunswick

Lewis, H (2000) *National Children's Bureau and the Council for Disabled Children's joint response to the Consultation Document: Promoting Health for Looked After Children: a guide to health care planning, assessment and monitoring.* National Children's Bureau (unpublished)

Lewis, H (1999) *Improving the Health of Children and Young People in Public Care: a manual for training residential social workers and foster carers*. National Children's Bureau

MacDonald, J (1993) *Primary Health Care: Medicine in its place*. Earthscan

McCann, J B and others (1996) Prevalence of psychiatric disorders in young people in the care system, *British Medical Journal*, 313, 1529-1530

McGuire, C and Corlyon, J (1997) *Health Promotion and Looked After Children in Brent and Harrow*. National Children's Bureau

Mather, M (2000a) Health issues for black and minority ethnic children, *Adoption and Fostering*, 24, 1, 68-70

Mather, M (2000b) Health needs of looked after children, *Children's Residential Care Unit Newsletter*, 13, (Spring), 3-4

Mather, M and Batty, D (2000) *Doctors for Children in Public Care. Advocating, promoting and protecting health*. British Agencies for Adoption and Fostering

Ministerial Task Force on Children's Safeguards (1998) *The Government's Response to the Children's Safeguards Review*. Stationery Office.

Morris, J (1999) *Hurtling Into a Void: Transition to adulthood for young disabled people with complex health and support needs*. Pavilion

Morris, J (1995) *Gone Missing: a research and policy review of disabled children living away from their families*. Who Cares? Trust

Naidoo, J and Wills, J (1994) *Health Promotion: Foundations for practice*. Bailliere Tindall Ltd

Petrie, P (2001) *A survey of pedagogy in Europe*. Unpublished report

Polnay, L (2000) Promoting the health of looked after children. Government proposals demand leadership and a culture change, *British Medical Journal*, 320,(11 March), 661-2

Richardson, J and Joughin C (2000) *The Mental Health Needs of Looked After Children*. Gaskell Publications

Rivers, K and others (1999) *Learning Lessons: a report on two research studies informing the National Healthy School Standard*. DoH and DfEE

Roberts, H (2000) *What Works in Reducing Inequalities in Child Health*. Barnardo's

Robbins, D (2000) *Tracking Progress in Children's Services: an evaluation of local responses to the Quality Protects Programme. Year 2 National Overview Report*. DoH

Saunders, L and Broad, B (1997) *The Health Needs of Young People Leaving Care*. De Montfort University

Save the Children (1995) *Does Anybody Care? Young people's research on leaving care*. (video) Save the Children

Seedhouse, D (1986) *Health: The foundations for achievement*. Wiley

Shaw, C and Who Cares? Trust (1998) *Remember My Messages*. Who Cares? Trust

Simard, Vachon and Berube *mentioned in* Kufeldt, K and others (2000) *Looking After Children in Canada*. University of New Brunswick

Simms (1991) *mentioned in* Kufeldt, K and others (2000) *Looking After Children in Canada*. University of New Brunswick

Skuse, T and Ward, H (1999) *Current Research Findings About the Health of Looked After Children. Paper for Quality Protects seminar: Improving Health Outcomes for Looked After Children, 6 December 1999*. Dartington Social Research Unit and Loughborough University

Support Force for Children's Residential Care (1995) *Good Care Matters: Ways of enhancing good practice in residential care*. DoH

Utting, W and others (1997) *People Like Us: The report of the review of the safeguards for children living away from home*. DoH

Varnava, G (1999) *Towards a Non-violent Society: Checkpoints for schools*. National Children's Bureau

Ward, H and Skuse, T (2001) *Looking After Children – transforming data into management information. Report from the first year of data collection*. DoH

West, A (1995) *You're on Your Own: Young people's research on leaving care*. Save the Children

World Health Organisation (1987) *Ottawa Charter, First International Conference on Health Promotion*. World Health Organisation: Ottawa

World Health Organisation (1946) *Constitution*. World Health Organisation: Geneva

Wyler, S (2000) *The Health of Young People Leaving Care: a review for the King's Fund/Oak Foundation*. King's Fund